30+

Fitness

Formula

Essential Exercises for Optimal Health and Vitality

BY SAM ABABIO

DEDICATION

To all those who believe in the power of perseverance and the pursuit of a healthier life, this book is for you.

To my family and friends, whose unwavering support and encouragement have always inspired me to reach for my goals.

And to everyone over 30 who is committed to embracing fitness and well-being, may this book be a guiding light on your journey to a stronger, healthier you.

Table of Contents

Introduction

Welcome to the 30+ Fitness Formula

Welcome to "30+ Fitness Formula: Essential Exercises for Optimal Health and Vitality." Whether you are just beginning your fitness journey or looking to refine your routine, this book aims to provide you with practical, effective exercises that are specifically tailored for those over 30. As we age, our bodies change, and so do our fitness needs. This guide will help you navigate these changes and maintain a healthy, active lifestyle.

Chapter 1: Understanding Fitness Over 30

As we age, maintaining physical fitness becomes increasingly important. This chapter will explore the physiological changes that occur after 30, including decreased muscle mass, reduced bone density, and slower metabolism. Understanding these changes is crucial for tailoring your fitness routine to ensure it remains effective and safe.

CHAPTER 2: Warm-Up Essentials

Before diving into your workout, it's essential to prepare your body with a proper warm-up. This chapter will cover the importance of warming up and provide a detailed guide to dynamic stretches and movements that increase blood flow and reduce the risk of injury.

Key Exercises:

1. Arm Circles

Purpose: Warm up the shoulder joints and increase flexibility.

How to Take Action:
Step 1: Take a straight stance and place your feet shoulder-width apart. Stretch your arms out to the sides, making a T shape with your body, so that they are parallel to the ground.
Start with Small Circles: Move your arms in small, controlled circles. Make a circle and move them forward. Make sure your movements are fluid and your arms are straight.
Enlarge the Circle: Make the circles bigger with each revolution by increasing their size gradually. For ten to fifteen seconds, keep doing this.
Forward Circles Completed: Now reverse the direction and begin creating backward circles. Once more, start out small and work your way up to larger circles.

Tips:

- Keep your movements controlled to avoid straining your shoulders.
- Engage your core to maintain balance.
- Ensure your shoulders stay down and relaxed, not hunched up towards your ears.

2. Leg Swings Leg Swings

Purpose: Loosen up the hip joints and increase flexibility in the legs and hips.

How to Perform:

1. **Starting Position:** Stand upright next to a wall or a sturdy object for support. Place one hand on the wall to maintain balance.
2. **Forward and Backward Swings:**
    - Shift your weight onto your left leg and swing your right leg forward and backward in a controlled manner.
    - Start with small swings and gradually increase the range of motion.
    - Keep your torso upright and avoid leaning forward or backward.
    - Perform 10-15 swings forward and backward on each leg.
3. **Side-to-Side Swings:**
    - Face the wall or support, and hold onto it with both hands.
    - Swing your right leg to the side and then across your body in front of your left leg.
    - Keep the swings controlled and increase the range of motion gradually.
    - Perform 10-15 side-to-side swings on each leg.

Tips:

- Keep your core engaged to maintain balance.
- Focus on smooth, controlled movements rather than speed.
- Make sure your standing leg remains slightly bent to avoid locking the knee.

3. Torso Twists

Purpose: Improve flexibility and mobility in the spine and torso.

How to Perform:

1. **Starting Position:** Stand with your feet shoulder-width apart and your knees slightly bent. Extend your arms out to the sides at shoulder height, parallel to the floor.
2. **Twisting Motion:**
    - Rotate your torso to the right, bringing your left arm across your body while keeping your hips facing forward.
    - Then, twist to the left, bringing your right arm across your body.
    - Continue twisting from side to side in a controlled manner.
3. **Controlled Movements:** Make sure the twist comes from your torso and not just your arms. Keep your hips stable and facing forward throughout the exercise.
4. **Breathing:** Exhale as you twist to each side and inhale as you return to the center.
5. **Duration:** Perform the torso twists for about 1-2 minutes, or 20-30 twists on each side.

Tips:

- Engage your core muscles to support your spine.
- Keep your movements slow and controlled to avoid any strain.
- Focus on the range of motion rather than speed to improve flexibility.

These exercises are great for warming up and improving flexibility, helping to prepare your body for more intense workouts or daily activities.

CHAPTER 3: Core Strength and Stability

A strong core is the foundation of overall fitness. It improves posture, reduces the risk of injury, and enhances balance. This chapter will detail essential core exercises, complete with step-by-step instructions and illustrations.

Key Exercises:

1. Plank

Purpose: The plank is an excellent core-strengthening exercise that also works the shoulders, arms, and glutes.

Steps:

1. **Starting Position:**
    - Begin on your hands and knees on a comfortable, flat surface like a yoga mat.
    - Place your forearms on the ground with your elbows directly under your shoulders. Your arms should form a 90-degree angle.
2. **Body Position:**
    - Extend your legs behind you, keeping your toes on the ground.
    - Engage your core muscles to lift your body into a straight line from your head to your heels. Your body should be in a straight line, not sagging or arching.
    - Your head should be in a neutral position, looking at the floor.
3. **Holding the Position:**
    - Keep your core tight and hold this position for as long as you can while maintaining proper form.
    - Breathe steadily and deeply throughout the exercise.
4. **Finishing the Exercise:**
    - Slowly lower your body back to the starting position on your hands and knees.

Tips:

- Keep your back flat and avoid letting your hips sag or rise.
- Focus on engaging your abdominal muscles to maintain stability.

- Start with shorter durations and gradually increase the time as you build strength.

Common Mistakes:

- Letting the hips drop or rise.
- Not engaging the core, leading to lower back strain.
- Holding the breath instead of breathing steadily.

2. Russian Twist

Purpose: The Russian twist is a core exercise that targets the obliques, helping to improve rotational strength and stability.

Steps:

1. **Starting Position:**
   - Sit on the floor with your knees bent and feet flat on the ground.
   - Lean back slightly so your torso is at about a 45-degree angle to the floor. Ensure your back is straight.
2. **Body Position:**
   - Clasp your hands together in front of your chest. For an added challenge, you can hold a weight or a medicine ball.
3. **Performing the Twist:**
   - Engage your core muscles and twist your torso to the right, bringing your clasped hands or the weight beside your hip.
   - Return to the center and then twist to the left, bringing your hands or the weight beside your left hip.
   - Continue alternating sides, twisting from the waist and not just moving your arms.
4. **Maintaining the Position:**
   - Keep your feet on the ground for stability. For an advanced variation, you can lift your feet off the ground, balancing on your sit bones.

Tips:

- Keep your movements controlled and deliberate to maximize muscle engagement.
- Focus on twisting your torso and engaging your obliques rather than just moving your arms.
- Breathe steadily throughout the exercise.

Common Mistakes:

- Rounding the back instead of keeping it straight.
- Using momentum to swing the arms instead of engaging the core to twist.
- Letting the feet lift off the ground unintentionally if you're keeping them grounded.

CHAPTER 4: Upper Body Strength

Building upper body strength is crucial for daily activities and overall fitness. This chapter focuses on exercises that target the chest, shoulders, back, and arms.

Key Exercises:

1. Push – up

How to Do a Push-Up

Description: A push-up is a classic upper body exercise that targets the chest, shoulders, triceps, and core. It's a great compound movement for building strength and muscle endurance.

Steps:

1. **Starting Position:**

- o Begin by lying face down on the floor. Position your hands slightly wider than shoulder-width apart.
  - o Your feet should be together, or you can place them slightly apart for better balance.
  - o Engage your core to keep your body in a straight line from head to heels.

2. **Body Position:**
   - o Your hands should be aligned with your chest, not your shoulders.
   - o Keep your fingers spread wide for better stability.
   - o Your neck should be in a neutral position, looking down at the floor.

3. **Lowering Phase:**
   - o Bend your elbows and lower your body toward the floor.
   - o Keep your elbows at about a 45-degree angle from your body, rather than flaring them out to the sides.
   - o Lower your body until your chest is just above the floor, or as far as you can go without compromising form.

4. **Pressing Phase:**
   - o Push through your palms to straighten your arms and lift your body back to the starting position.
   - o Make sure to keep your core engaged to maintain a straight body line.
   - o Avoid locking your elbows at the top of the movement.

5. **Breathing:**
   - o Inhale as you lower your body toward the floor.
   - o Exhale as you push back up to the starting position.

6. **Repetition:**
   - o Repeat for the desired number of repetitions, maintaining proper form throughout each rep.

Common Mistakes:

- Letting your hips sag or pike.
- Flaring your elbows out to the sides.

- Not maintaining a straight line from head to heels.

Modifications:

- **Knee Push-Ups:** Perform the push-up with your knees on the floor for less resistance.
- **Elevated Push-Ups:** Place your hands on an elevated surface like a bench or step to reduce difficulty.

2. **Dumbbell Row**

How to Do a Dumbbell Row

Description: The dumbbell row is an effective exercise for targeting the upper back, including the latissimus dorsi, rhomboids, and trapezius muscles. It also engages the biceps and forearms.

Steps:

1. **Starting Position:**
   - Stand with your feet shoulder-width apart, holding a dumbbell in each hand.
   - Bend your knees slightly and hinge at your hips, pushing your butt back as if you were about to sit down.
   - Keep your back straight and your torso inclined at about a 45-degree angle to the floor.
   - Let the dumbbells hang at arm's length from your shoulders, with your palms facing each other.
2. **Body Position:**
   - Engage your core to stabilize your spine.
   - Maintain a neutral neck position by looking a few feet in front of you on the floor.
3. **Rowing Phase:**
   - Pull the dumbbells towards your torso by bending your elbows and squeezing your shoulder blades together.

- o Keep your elbows close to your body, rather than flaring them out to the sides.
- o Continue pulling until the dumbbells are level with your ribcage.

4. **Lowering Phase:**
   - o Slowly lower the dumbbells back to the starting position, fully extending your arms.
   - o Keep your back straight and your core engaged throughout the movement.
5. **Breathing:**
   - o Inhale as you lower the dumbbells.
   - o Exhale as you pull the dumbbells towards your torso.
6. **Repetition:**
   - o Repeat for the desired number of repetitions, maintaining proper form throughout each rep.

Common Mistakes:

- Rounding or arching the back.
- Using momentum to lift the weights.
- Letting the elbows flare out too much.

Modifications:

- **Single-Arm Dumbbell Row:** Perform the exercise one arm at a time, placing your free hand on a bench for support.
- **Supported Dumbbell Row:** Rest your non-working hand and knee on a bench for added stability and focus on form.

CHAPTER 5: Lower Body Strength

Strong legs are essential for mobility and stability. This chapter highlights exercises that focus on the quadriceps, hamstrings, glutes, and calves.

<u>**Key Exercises:**</u>

1. Squats

Purpose: Squats primarily target the quadriceps, hamstrings, glutes, and core muscles.

How to Perform a Squat:

1. **Starting Position:**
   - Stand with your feet shoulder-width apart.
   - Keep your toes pointed slightly outward.
   - Engage your core and keep your chest up.
   - Place your hands on your hips, or extend them straight out in front of you for balance.
2. **Lowering Phase:**
   - Begin the movement by pushing your hips back as if you are sitting down in a chair.
   - Bend your knees and lower your body, keeping your weight on your heels.
   - Continue to lower until your thighs are at least parallel to the ground (or as low as your mobility allows).
3. **Form Tips:**
   - Keep your back straight and chest up throughout the movement.
   - Make sure your knees do not extend beyond your toes.
   - Keep your knees in line with your toes (don't let them cave inward).
4. **Rising Phase:**
   - Push through your heels to return to the starting position.
   - Straighten your legs and extend your hips fully.
   - Squeeze your glutes at the top of the movement.
5. **Breathing:**
   - Inhale as you lower into the squat.
   - Exhale as you push back up to standing.

Common Mistakes to Avoid:

- **Letting your knees cave inward:** Keep them aligned with your toes.
- **Rounding your back:** Maintain a neutral spine throughout the movement.
- **Lifting your heels:** Keep your heels grounded to maintain balance and proper form.

2. Lunges

Purpose: Lunges target the quadriceps, hamstrings, glutes, and calves. They also help improve balance and coordination.

How to Perform a Lunge:

1. **Starting Position:**
   - Stand with your feet hip-width apart.
   - Engage your core and keep your chest up.
   - Place your hands on your hips or hold them out to the sides for balance.
2. **Stepping Phase:**
   - Take a step forward with your right foot.
   - Lower your body by bending both knees to create two 90-degree angles with your legs.
3. **Lowering Phase:**
   - Your right thigh should be parallel to the ground and your right knee should be directly above your ankle.
   - Your left knee should hover just above the ground (or lightly touch if needed).
4. **Form Tips:**
   - Keep your upper body straight and your core engaged.
   - Ensure your front knee does not extend beyond your toes.
   - Your back heel should be lifted off the ground.
5. **Rising Phase:**

- Push through the heel of your front foot to return to the starting position.
  - Bring your right foot back to meet your left foot.
6. **Alternating Legs:**
  - Repeat the movement with your left leg stepping forward.
7. **Breathing:**
  - Inhale as you lower into the lunge.
  - Exhale as you push back up to standing.

Common Mistakes to Avoid:

- **Allowing your front knee to go past your toes:** This can place undue stress on your knee.
- **Leaning forward:** Keep your torso upright to maintain balance and proper form.
- **Not stepping far enough:** Ensure a big enough step to create two 90-degree angles in your legs.

CHAPTER 6: Cardio for Heart Health

Cardiovascular exercise is vital for maintaining heart health and overall fitness. This chapter provides effective cardio workouts that can be done at home or in the gym.

Key Exercises:

1. **Jump Rope**

Overview: Jump rope is a highly effective cardiovascular exercise that improves coordination, agility, and overall fitness. It engages multiple muscle groups, including the calves, quads, hamstrings, glutes, and shoulders.

Step-by-Step Instructions:

1. **Equipment Needed:**
   - A jump rope suitable for your height.
   - Comfortable athletic shoes with good support.
   - An open space with a flat surface to avoid tripping.
2. **Setup:**
   - Adjust the jump rope length: Step on the middle of the rope with one foot. The handles should reach up to your armpits when pulled taut.
   - Stand with your feet together and hold the rope handles at your sides.
3. **Starting Position:**
   - Hold the handles with a firm grip.
   - Keep your elbows close to your body, with your forearms parallel to the ground.
   - Stand upright with a slight bend in your knees.
4. **The Jump:**
   - Swing the rope over your head using your wrists, not your arms.
   - Jump just high enough for the rope to pass under your feet (about 1-2 inches off the ground).
   - Land softly on the balls of your feet with knees slightly bent to absorb the impact.
5. **Rhythm and Breathing:**
   - Maintain a consistent rhythm; try to keep your jumps smooth and controlled.
   - Breathe steadily, exhaling on the jump and inhaling as the rope swings overhead.
6. **Common Variations:**
   - **Basic Jump:** Both feet leave the ground and land simultaneously.
   - **Alternate Foot Jump:** Jump from one foot to the other, like running in place.
   - **High Knees Jump:** Incorporate a high knee raise with each jump for added intensity.
7. **Safety Tips:**

- o Ensure the jump rope is not too long or too short.
- o Avoid jumping on hard surfaces to reduce joint impact.
- o Warm up before starting and cool down after completing your session.

3. High Knees

Overview: High knees is a dynamic exercise that boosts cardiovascular endurance, strengthens the lower body, and engages the core. It mimics running in place with exaggerated knee lifts.

Step-by-Step Instructions:

1. **Setup:**
   - o No equipment is required, just comfortable athletic shoes.
   - o Perform the exercise in an open space with a flat, non-slip surface.
2. **Starting Position:**
   - o Stand with your feet hip-width apart.
   - o Keep your back straight and engage your core muscles.
   - o Place your hands in front of you at waist height, palms facing down.
3. **The Movement:**
   - o Lift your right knee as high as possible towards your chest, ideally above hip level.
   - o Quickly switch and lift your left knee as high as possible while lowering your right leg.
   - o Continue alternating legs at a rapid pace, like running in place with exaggerated knee lifts.
4. **Arm Motion:**
   - o Swing your arms naturally, as if you were running. Alternatively, you can keep your hands at waist height and aim to tap your knees to your palms.
5. **Rhythm and Breathing:**
   - o Maintain a steady rhythm, aiming for a quick and consistent pace.

- o Breathe rhythmically, exhaling with each knee lift and inhaling as you switch legs.
6. **Intensity Modifications:**
   - o **Beginner:** Start with a slower pace and lower knee lifts, gradually increasing speed and height.
   - o **Advanced:** Incorporate arm movements or perform the exercise on a slightly elevated surface.
7. **Safety Tips:**
   - o Land softly on the balls of your feet to minimize impact on your joints.
   - o Keep your core engaged to maintain balance and stability.
   - o Avoid leaning back or forward; keep your torso upright throughout the exercise.
8. **Common Variations:**
   - o **High Knees with Arm Swings:** Swing your arms as if running.
   - o **High Knees with Twist:** Add a slight twist at the waist to engage the obliques.

CHAPTER 7: Flexibility and Mobility

Flexibility and mobility exercises help maintain joint health and reduce the risk of injury. This chapter includes essential stretches and movements to enhance flexibility.

Key Exercises:

1. **Forward Bend (Standing Forward Bend or Uttanasana)**

Description:

The Standing Forward Bend is a common yoga pose that stretches the hamstrings, calves, and lower back. It can help relieve stress and improve flexibility.

Steps:

1. **Starting Position**:
   - Stand tall with your feet hip-width apart and arms by your sides. Distribute your weight evenly across both feet.
2. **Inhale and Lengthen**:
   - Inhale deeply, and as you do so, stretch your arms overhead to lengthen your spine. Imagine creating space between each vertebra.
3. **Forward Bend**:
   - As you exhale, begin to hinge at your hips, not your waist, and slowly fold your torso forward. Keep your back straight initially as you bend.
4. **Reach Down**:
   - Allow your arms to hang down towards the floor, or if flexibility allows, place your hands on the floor, your shins, or hold onto your ankles. Let your head hang heavy, and relax your neck.
5. **Deepen the Stretch**:
   - If comfortable, you can gently pull yourself deeper into the stretch by engaging your core and drawing your chest closer to your legs. Keep your knees soft or slightly bent if you feel too much strain in your hamstrings.
6. **Hold the Pose**:
   - Breathe deeply and hold the pose for 15-30 seconds, or longer if comfortable. Focus on releasing tension in your back and legs with each exhale.
7. **Return to Standing**:

- To come out of the pose, engage your core and slowly roll your spine up to standing, vertebra by vertebra. Your head should be the last to come up. Inhale as you raise your arms overhead again, and exhale as you bring them back to your sides.

Tips:

- Keep a slight bend in your knees to avoid over-stretching your hamstrings.
- Use a yoga block or place your hands on your thighs if you can't reach the floor.
- Keep your movements slow and controlled to prevent dizziness or strain.

2. Cat-Cow Stretch (Marjaryasana-Bitilasana)

Description:

The Cat-Cow Stretch is a gentle flow between two poses that warms up the spine and relieves tension in the back and neck. It's excellent for improving flexibility and promoting spinal health.

Steps:

1. **Starting Position**:
   - Begin on your hands and knees in a tabletop position. Ensure your wrists are directly under your shoulders and your knees are under your hips. Keep your head in a neutral position, eyes looking at the floor.
2. **Cat Pose (Marjaryasana)**:
   - As you exhale, round your spine towards the ceiling. Tuck your tailbone under, draw your belly button towards your spine, and drop your head, bringing your chin towards your chest. Feel the stretch along your entire back.
3. **Cow Pose (Bitilasana)**:

- o   As you inhale, arch your back by lifting your sitting bones and chest towards the ceiling. Let your belly drop towards the floor. Lift your head and gaze straight ahead or slightly upwards, without straining your neck.
4. **Flow Between the Poses**:
   - o   Continue to flow between Cat and Cow poses, syncing your breath with your movements. Inhale as you move into Cow pose, and exhale as you transition into Cat pose.
5. **Repeat the Sequence**:
   - o   Perform the sequence for 5-10 breaths, or as long as feels good. Focus on smooth, continuous movements and deep, rhythmic breathing.

Tips:

- Move slowly and mindfully, especially if you have any back or neck issues.
- Keep your arms straight but not locked, with your shoulder blades moving apart in Cat pose and together in Cow pose.
- Ensure that your movements are controlled and that you're not straining your back or neck.

CHAPTER 8: Balance and Coordination

Improving balance and coordination is crucial for preventing falls and enhancing overall fitness. This chapter covers exercises that target these areas.

Key Exercises:

1. Single Leg Stand

Purpose: The single leg stand exercise improves balance, stability, and strengthens the muscles of the legs, hips, and core.

Steps:

1. **Starting Position:**
   - Stand upright with your feet hip-width apart.
   - Place your hands on your hips or extend your arms out to your sides for balance.
2. **Lifting One Leg:**
   - Shift your weight onto your right foot.
   - Slowly lift your left foot off the ground, bending your knee to bring your left thigh parallel to the floor, or as high as is comfortable.
   - Maintain a straight posture and keep your core engaged.
3. **Balancing:**
   - Hold this position for 10-30 seconds, focusing on a point in front of you to help maintain balance.
   - If you feel unsteady, lightly touch a nearby wall or chair for support.
4. **Switching Legs:**
   - Slowly lower your left foot back to the ground.
   - Repeat the exercise on the opposite side by lifting your right foot off the ground.
5. **Repetitions:**
   - Perform 2-3 sets of 10-15 seconds on each leg, gradually increasing the duration as your balance improves.

Tips:

- Keep your standing knee slightly bent to avoid locking the joint.
- Engage your core muscles to help stabilize your body.
- Practice this exercise near a wall or sturdy chair if you're new to balance exercises.

2. Heel-to-Toe Walk

Purpose: The heel-to-toe walk is a simple exercise that improves balance, coordination, and lower body strength, which is particularly beneficial for fall prevention.

Steps:

1. **Starting Position:**
   - Stand upright with your feet together and your arms relaxed at your sides.
   - Find a straight path, like a hallway or a long room, to perform the exercise.
2. **Walking Forward:**
   - Lift your right foot and place your right heel directly in front of your left toe.
   - Shift your weight onto your right foot and lift your left foot, placing your left heel directly in front of your right toe.
3. **Maintaining Balance:**
   - Continue walking forward in a straight line, ensuring each step places your heel directly in front of your opposite toe.
   - Keep your eyes focused on a point ahead of you rather than looking down at your feet.
   - Use your arms for balance, extending them slightly out to your sides if needed.
4. **Reversing the Walk:**
   - Once you reach the end of your path, turn around carefully and repeat the heel-to-toe walk in the opposite direction.
5. **Repetitions:**
   - Perform the heel-to-toe walk for 10-15 steps in each direction, repeating for 2-3 sets.

Tips:

- Walk slowly and deliberately to maintain your balance.
- Engage your core muscles to help stabilize your body.
- If you feel unsteady, perform the exercise near a wall or have a sturdy object nearby to hold onto.

Both exercises are excellent for improving balance, coordination, and lower body strength, making them valuable additions to your fitness routine, especially as you age.

CHAPTER 9: Full-Body Workouts

Full-body workouts are efficient and effective for building strength and endurance. This chapter provides comprehensive exercises that engage multiple muscle groups.

Key Exercises:

1. Burpees

Description: Burpees are a full-body exercise that combines strength training and cardio. They target various muscle groups, including the chest, arms, quads, glutes, hamstrings, and core.

Step-by-Step Instructions:

1. **Start Position:**
   - Stand with your feet shoulder-width apart and your arms at your sides.
2. **Squat Down:**
   - Lower your body into a squat position by bending your knees and pushing your hips back. Place your hands on the floor in front of you, just inside your feet.
3. **Kick Back:**
   - Jump your feet back so that you are in a high plank position with your body forming a straight line from your head to your heels. Keep your core engaged to maintain stability.
4. **Push-Up (optional):**
   - Perform a push-up by bending your elbows and lowering your chest to the floor. Then push back up to return to the

plank position. This step can be skipped if you're a beginner or want a less intense variation.

5. **Jump Forward:**
   - Jump your feet forward to land just outside of your hands, returning to the squat position.
6. **Jump Up:**
   - Explosively jump up into the air, reaching your arms overhead. Land softly and immediately lower back into the squat position to begin the next rep.

Tips:

- Keep your movements fluid and controlled.
- Ensure your back stays straight and your core is engaged during the plank and push-up phases.
- Breathe steadily throughout the exercise, exhaling on the jump up.

2. Mountain Climbers

Description: Mountain climbers are a high-intensity exercise that engages multiple muscle groups, including the shoulders, arms, chest, core, and legs. They are excellent for building cardiovascular endurance, core strength, and agility.

Step-by-Step Instructions:

1. **Start Position:**
   - Begin in a high plank position with your hands directly under your shoulders and your body forming a straight line from head to heels. Keep your core tight.
2. **Drive One Knee Forward:**
   - Bring your right knee towards your chest, keeping your left leg extended. Your right foot should hover just above the ground.
3. **Switch Legs:**

- Quickly switch legs by extending your right leg back and bringing your left knee towards your chest. This movement should be fast and controlled, as if you are running in place.

4. **Continue Alternating:**
   - Continue alternating your legs, maintaining a steady rhythm. Your body should stay in a straight line, and your hips should remain low, avoiding any bouncing or lifting.

Tips:

- Keep your core engaged throughout the exercise to stabilize your body.
- Maintain a consistent pace that challenges you but allows you to maintain proper form.
- Breathe steadily, exhaling with each knee drive.

Combining Both Exercises in a Workout

To create an effective workout, you can alternate between burpees and mountain climbers. For example:

- Perform 10 burpees followed by 30 seconds of mountain climbers.
- Rest for 30-60 seconds.
- Repeat for 3-5 rounds.

This combination provides a high-intensity workout that targets multiple muscle groups and improves both strength and cardiovascular endurance.

CHAPTER 10: Recovery and Cool Down

Proper recovery and cool-down techniques are essential for preventing injury and promoting muscle recovery. This chapter includes gentle stretches and relaxation exercises.

Key Exercises:

1. Child's Pose (Balasana)

Purpose: The Child's Pose is a gentle stretch for the back, hips, thighs, and ankles. It helps to relieve tension and stress.

Steps:

1. **Start Position**:
   - Begin on your hands and knees in a tabletop position. Ensure your wrists are directly under your shoulders and your knees are under your hips.
2. **Lowering Down**:
   - Bring your big toes together and widen your knees towards the edges of your mat.
3. **Sitting Back**:
   - Slowly sit back onto your heels. As you do so, your hips will lower towards your feet. If your hips don't reach your feet comfortably, place a blanket or cushion between your thighs and calves for support.
4. **Extending Forward**:
   - Stretch your arms forward, placing your palms flat on the mat. Extend your arms as far as comfortable, feeling a gentle stretch along your back and arms. Alternatively, you can keep your arms alongside your body with palms facing up if that feels more relaxing.
5. **Resting Position**:
   - Lower your forehead to the mat. If this is uncomfortable, you can place a block or a folded blanket under your forehead for support.
6. **Breathing**:
   - Take slow, deep breaths. Inhale deeply, feeling your back expand, and exhale slowly, feeling your body sink deeper into the pose.
7. **Duration**:

- Stay in this position for as long as it feels comfortable, typically 1-3 minutes. Focus on relaxing and releasing any tension in your body.

8. **Returning to Start**:
   - To come out of the pose, gently lift your forehead and walk your hands back towards your knees. Slowly return to the tabletop position.

Tips:

- If you have knee issues, place a rolled-up blanket behind your knees for extra cushioning.
- Keep your eyes closed and focus on your breath to enhance relaxation.

2. Seated Forward Bend (Paschimottanasana)

Purpose: The Seated Forward Bend stretches the spine, shoulders, hamstrings, and calves. It calms the mind and relieves stress.

Steps:

1. **Start Position**:
   - Sit on the floor with your legs extended straight in front of you. Flex your feet so that your toes point towards the ceiling.
2. **Alignment**:
   - Sit up tall, lengthening your spine. If your lower back feels tight or you have difficulty sitting up straight, you can sit on a folded blanket or a yoga block for added height and support.
3. **Inhaling**:
   - Inhale deeply, raising your arms overhead to lengthen your spine further.
4. **Bending Forward**:

- As you exhale, hinge at your hips (not your waist) and begin to fold forward. Lead with your chest, aiming to keep your back as straight as possible.

5. **Reaching Forward**:
   - Reach your hands towards your feet, shins, or ankles—wherever they can comfortably reach without forcing. If you can, hold your feet and gently pull yourself a bit further into the stretch.

6. **Relaxing into the Stretch**:
   - Allow your torso to rest on your thighs as much as possible. If you can't reach your feet, you can use a strap around your feet to gently pull yourself forward.

7. **Breathing**:
   - Take deep, steady breaths. With each inhale, think about lengthening your spine, and with each exhale, think about deepening the fold.

8. **Holding the Pose**:
   - Stay in this position for 1-3 minutes, depending on your comfort level. Focus on releasing any tension and stretching gently.

9. **Returning to Start**:
   - To come out of the pose, engage your core, and slowly rise back up to a seated position as you inhale. Lower your arms back down to your sides.

Tips:

- Avoid rounding your back excessively. The goal is to stretch the spine and hamstrings, not to reach your feet at all costs.
- Keep your shoulders relaxed and away from your ears.
- Use props like yoga blocks or straps to make the pose more accessible if needed.

By practicing these exercises regularly, you can improve flexibility, reduce stress, and promote overall physical well-being.

Conclusion

Maintaining a balanced fitness routine is essential for achieving and sustaining overall health and well-being, especially as we age. The 30+ Fitness Formula offers a comprehensive approach to fitness, focusing on exercises that promote strength, flexibility, and cardiovascular health tailored for individuals over 30. By integrating these exercises into your daily routine, you can experience increased energy levels, reduced stress, and improved physical and mental health.

Consistency is key. Regular exercise not only enhances your immediate quality of life but also provides long-term benefits such as increased muscle mass, better joint mobility, and a stronger immune system. Staying committed to your fitness journey will help you age gracefully, maintain your independence, and enjoy an active lifestyle for years to come.

Remember, every step you take towards your fitness goals is a step towards a healthier, happier you. Embrace the 30+ Fitness Formula, stay motivated, and keep pushing forward. Your future self will thank you for the dedication and effort you invest today. Keep moving, stay strong, and enjoy the journey to a vibrant and fit life.

www.ingramcontent.com/pod-product-compliance
Lightning Source LLC
Chambersburg PA
CBHW081501250726
48662CB00009B/3176